I0845325

Sarah has Tourette's
(and it's okay)

written and illustrated by Kaitlyn Craig

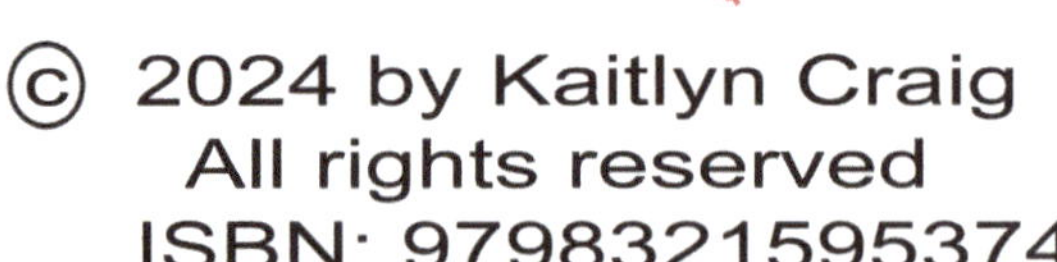

ISBN: 9798321595374

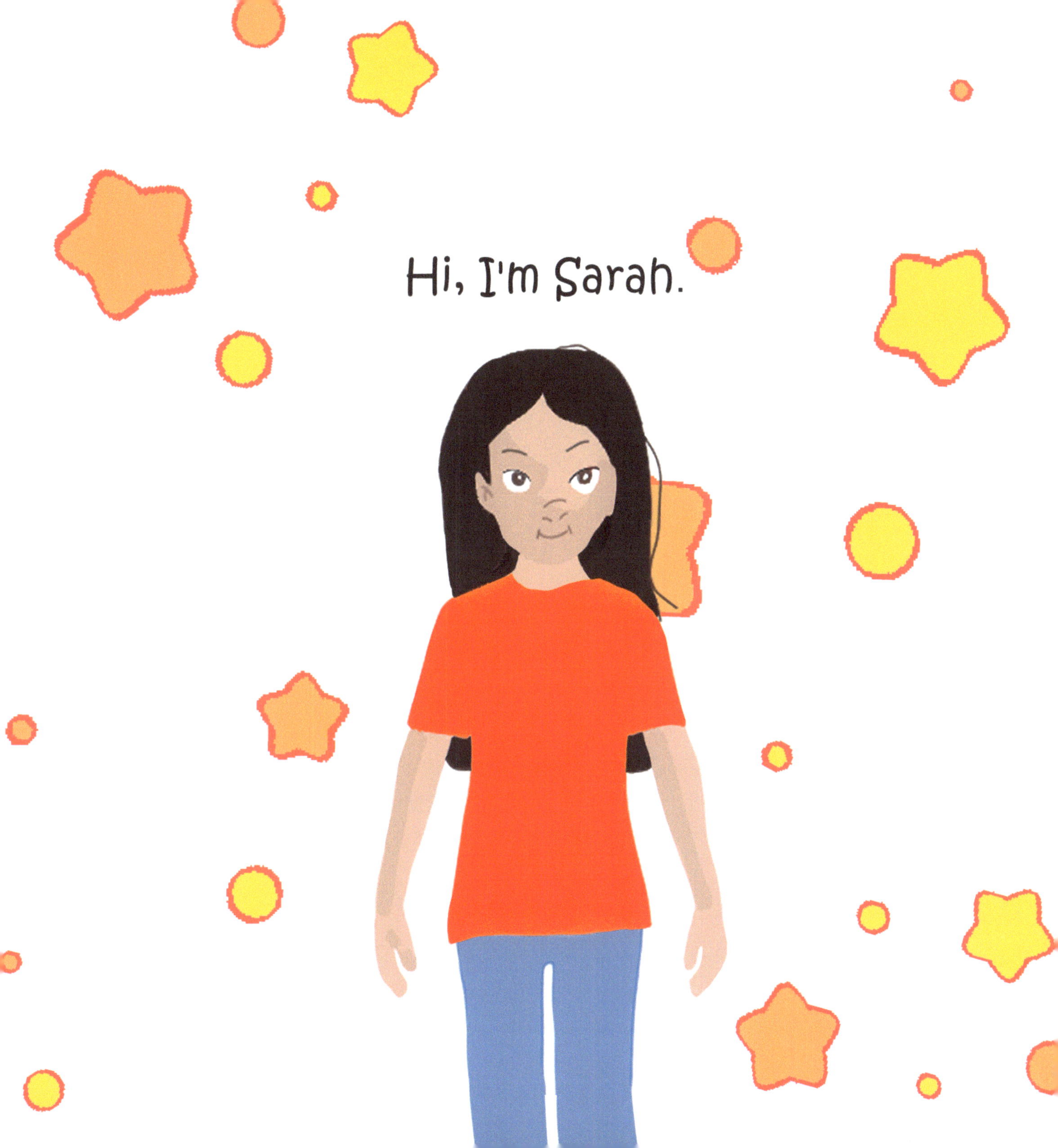
Hi, I'm Sarah.

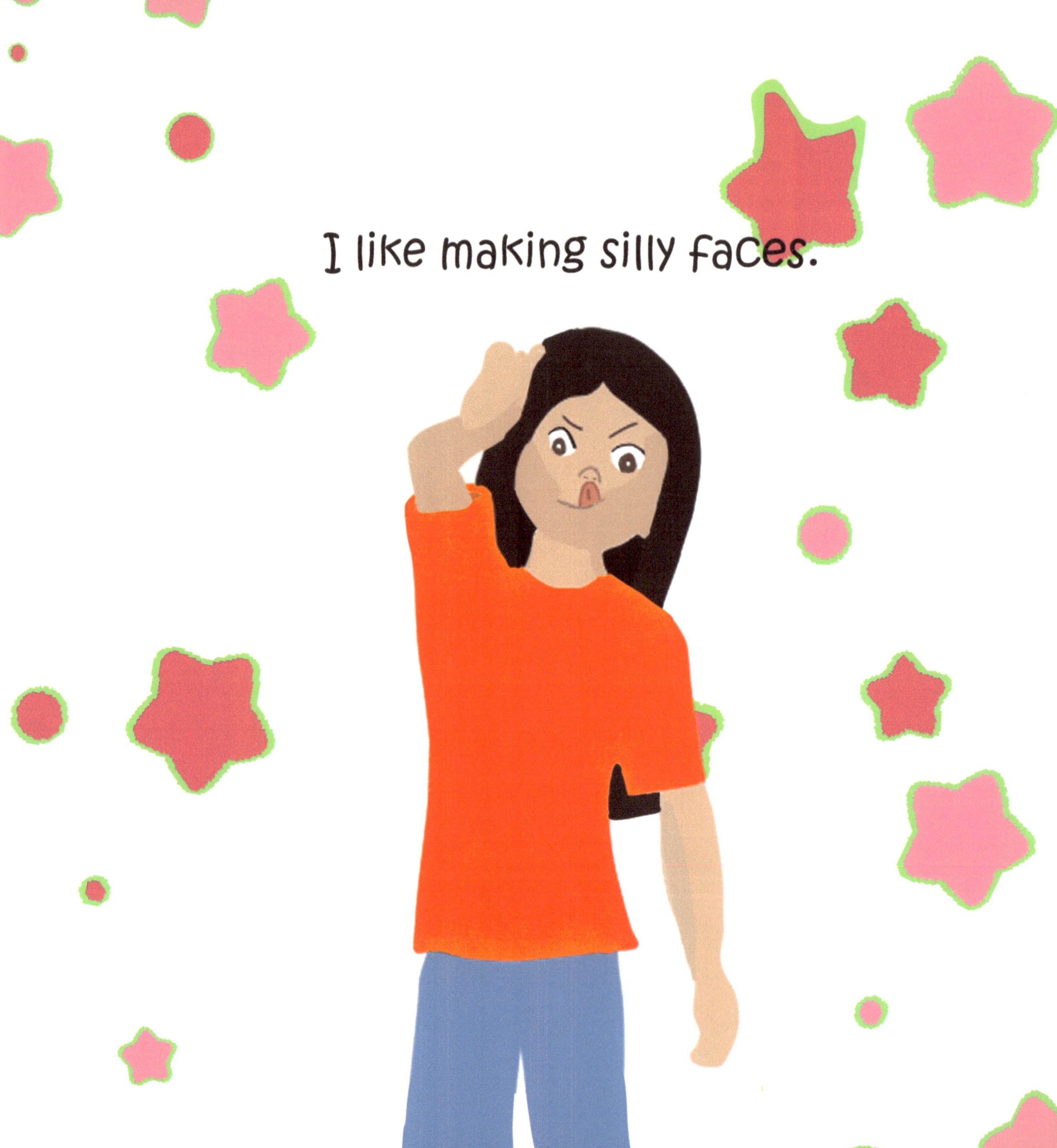
I like making silly faces.

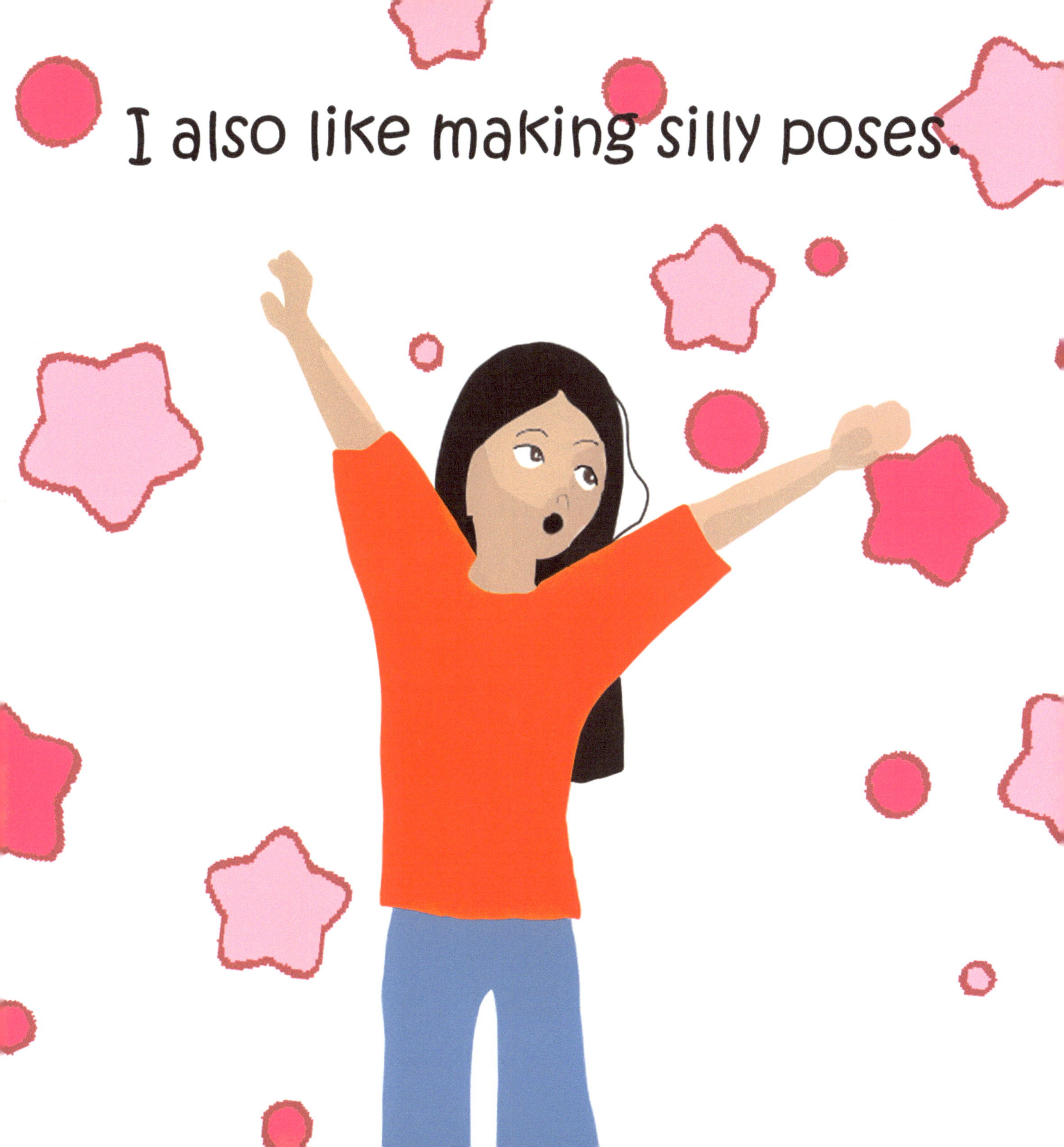I also like making silly poses.

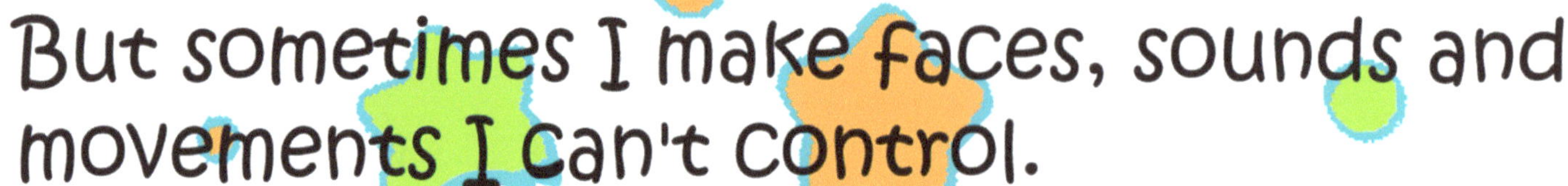
But sometimes I make faces, sounds and movements I can't control.

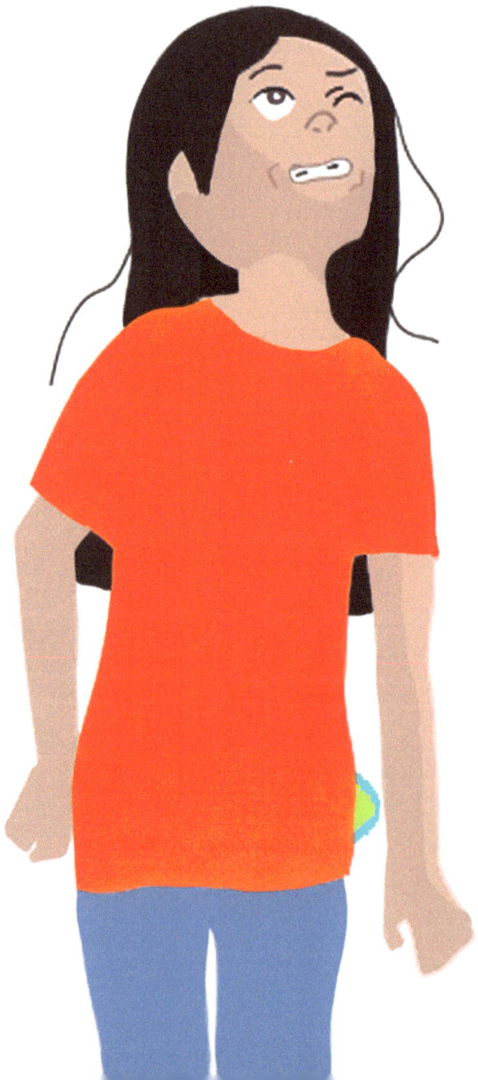

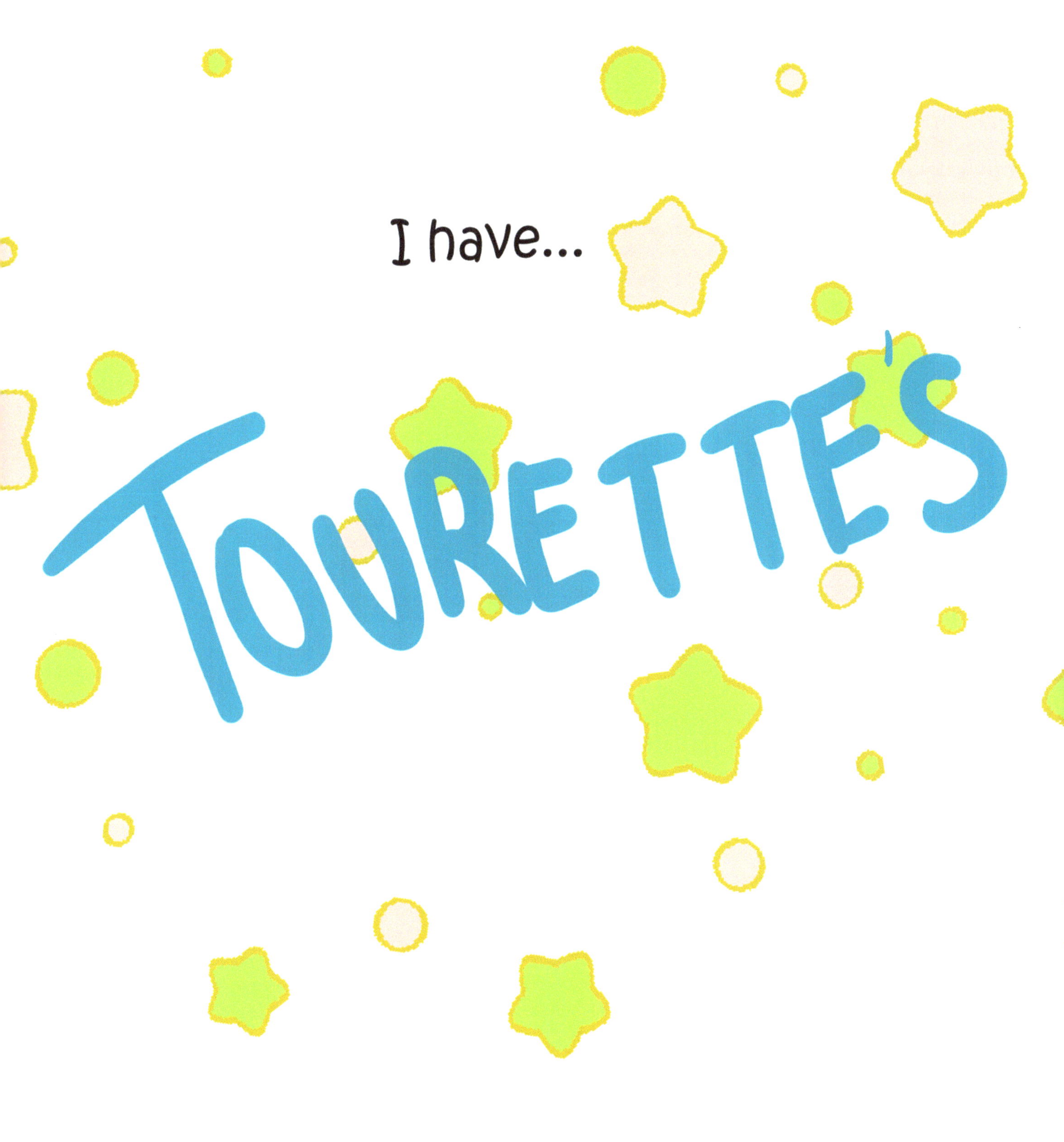
I have...
TOURETTE'S

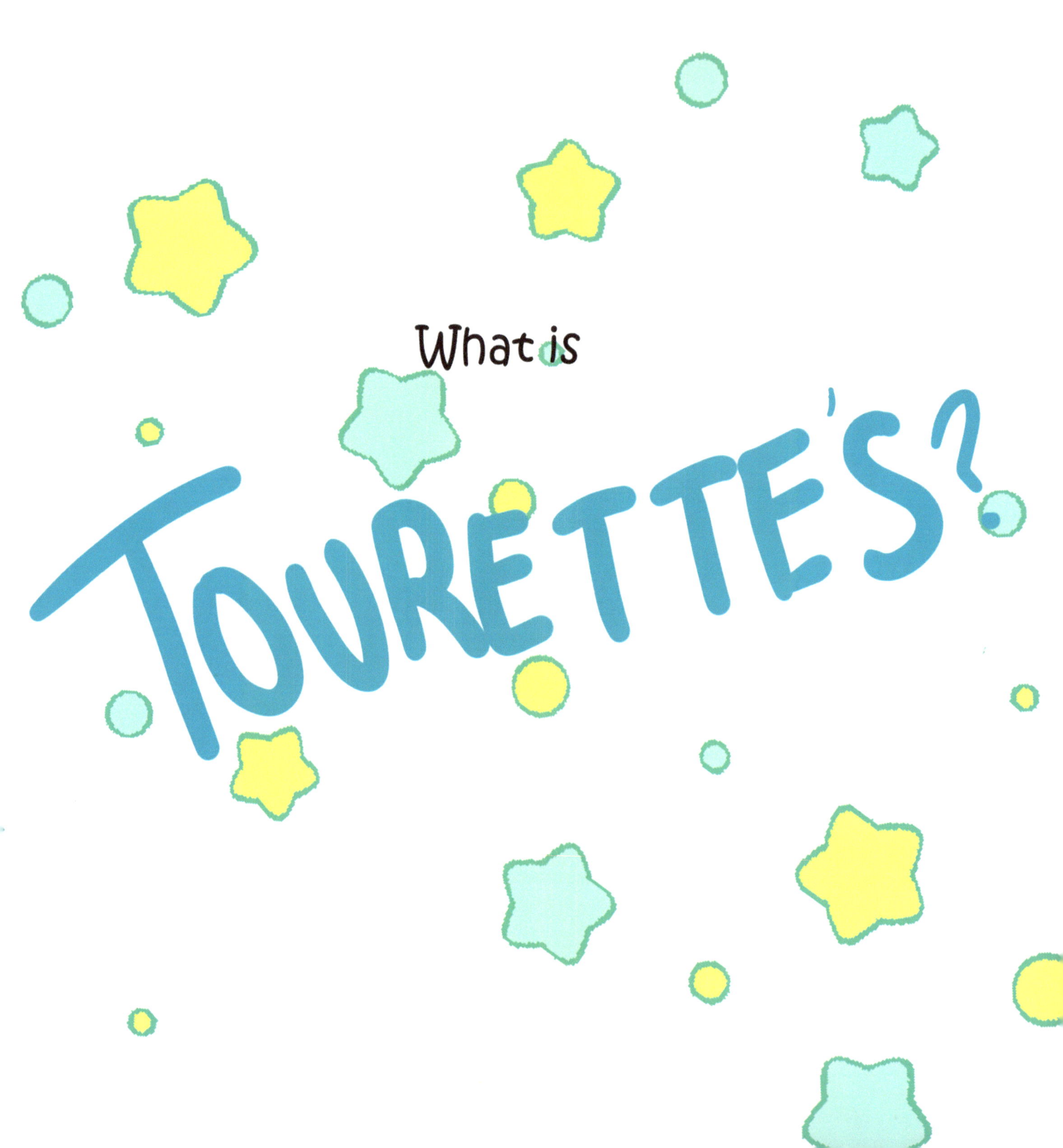

What is
TOURETTE'S?

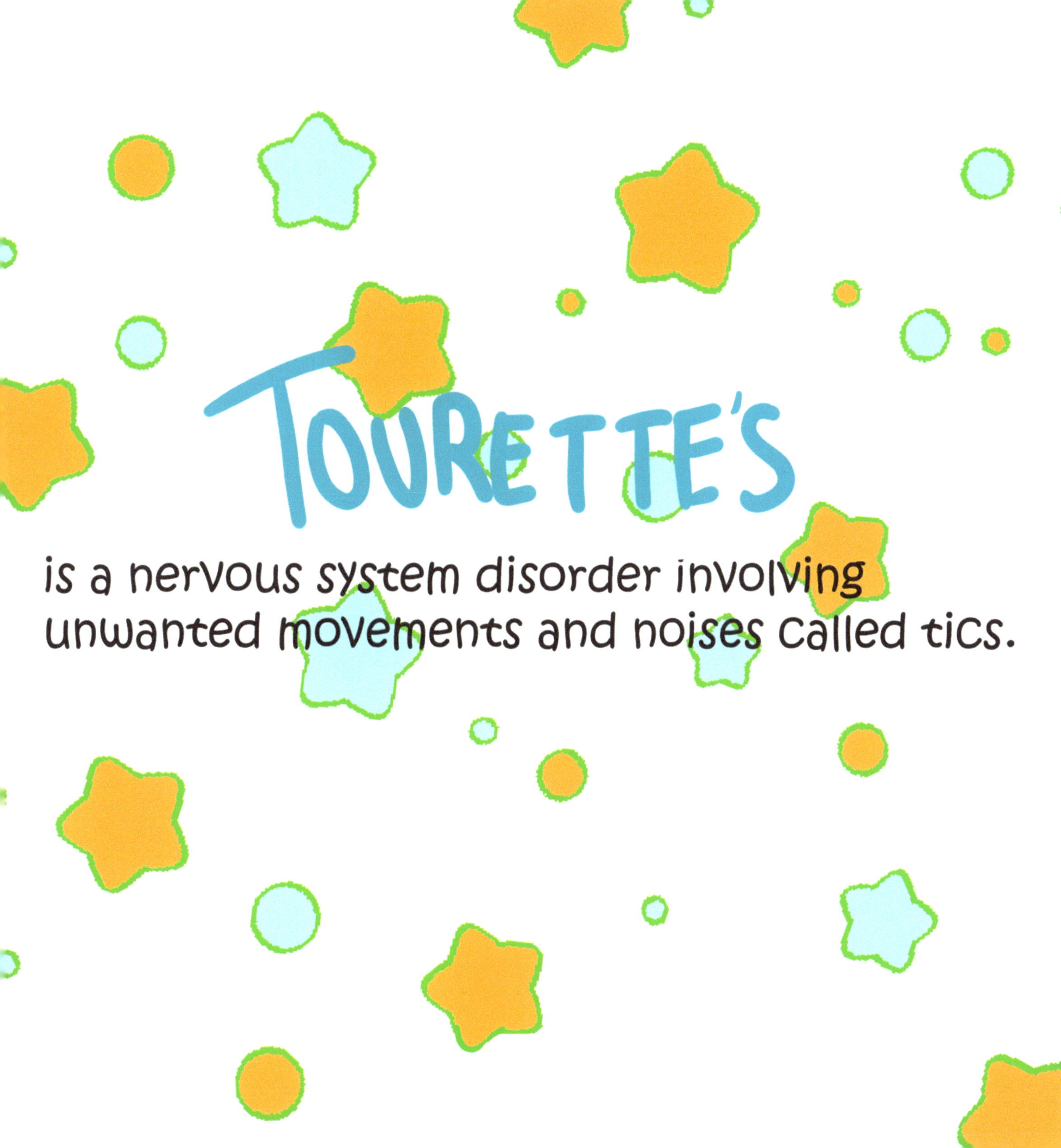

TOURETTE'S
is a nervous system disorder involving unwanted movements and noises called tics.

Shrugging

Blinking

Tics can include...

Tongue Clicking

Clapping

Repeated Phrases

grimacing

eye rolling

& more

But that doesn't mean everyone has the same tics. Tics differ in everyone.

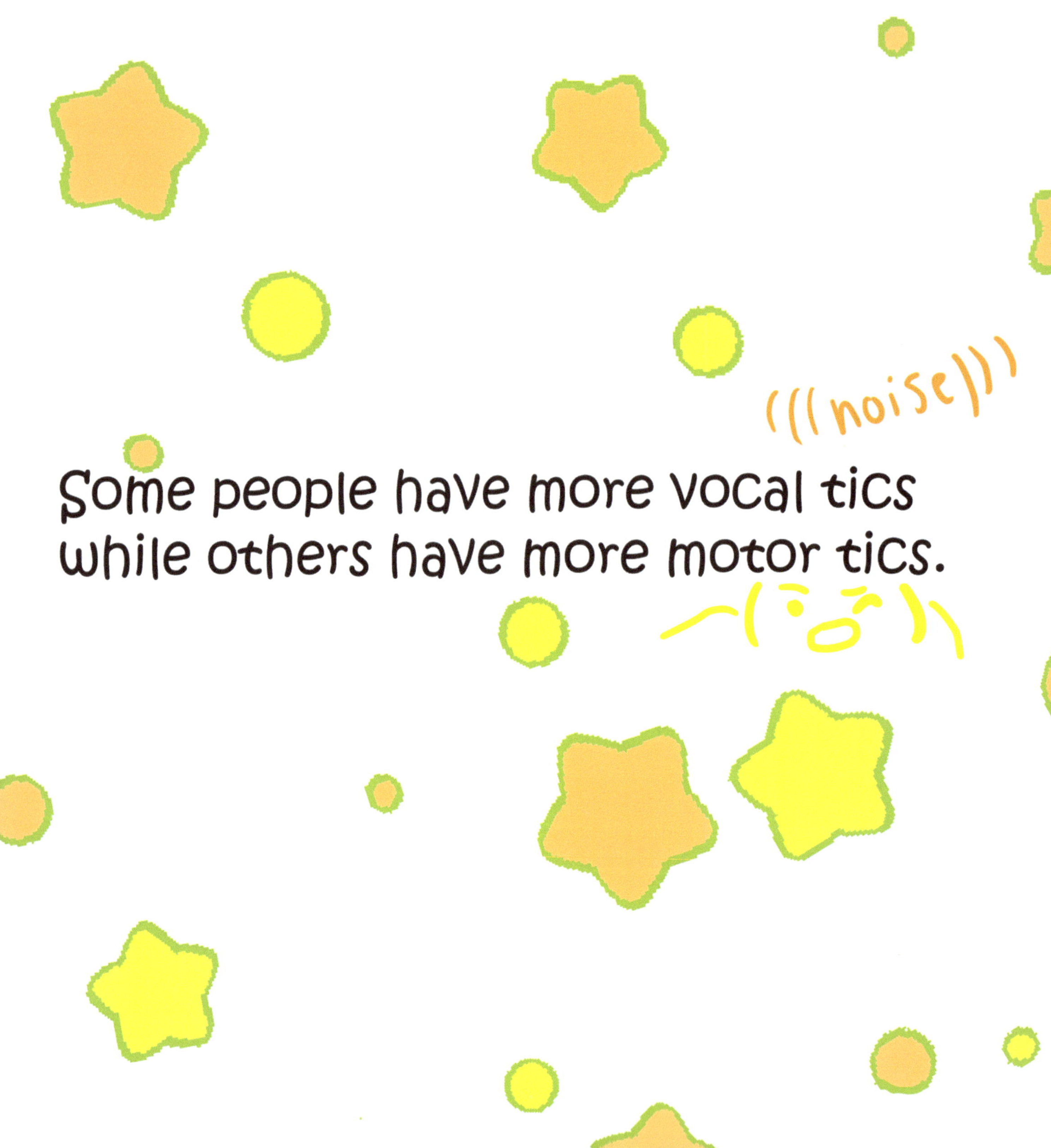
(((noise)))
Some people have more vocal tics
while others have more motor tics.
ヘ(˙□˙)ﾉ

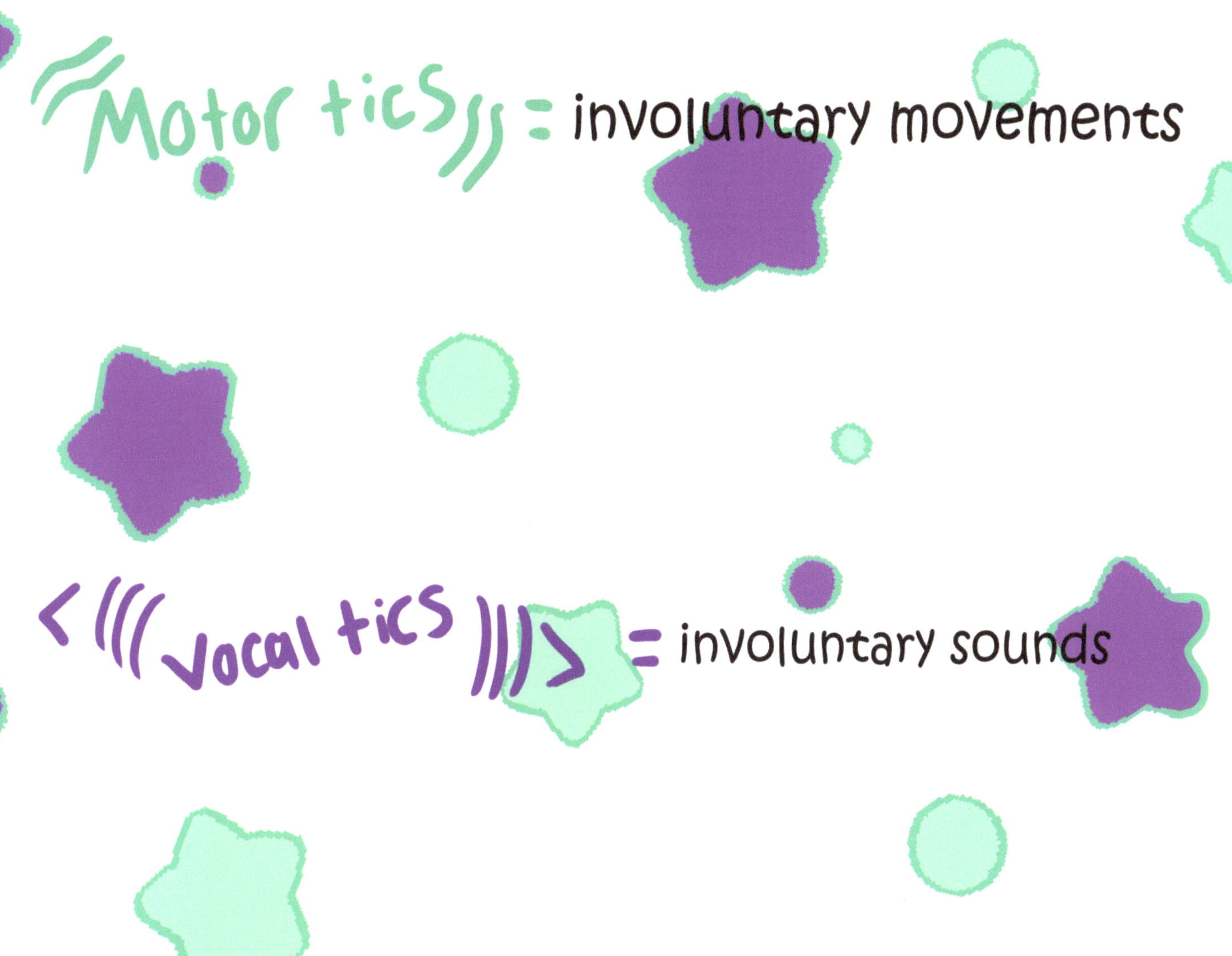
Motor tics = involuntary movements
vocal tics = involuntary sounds

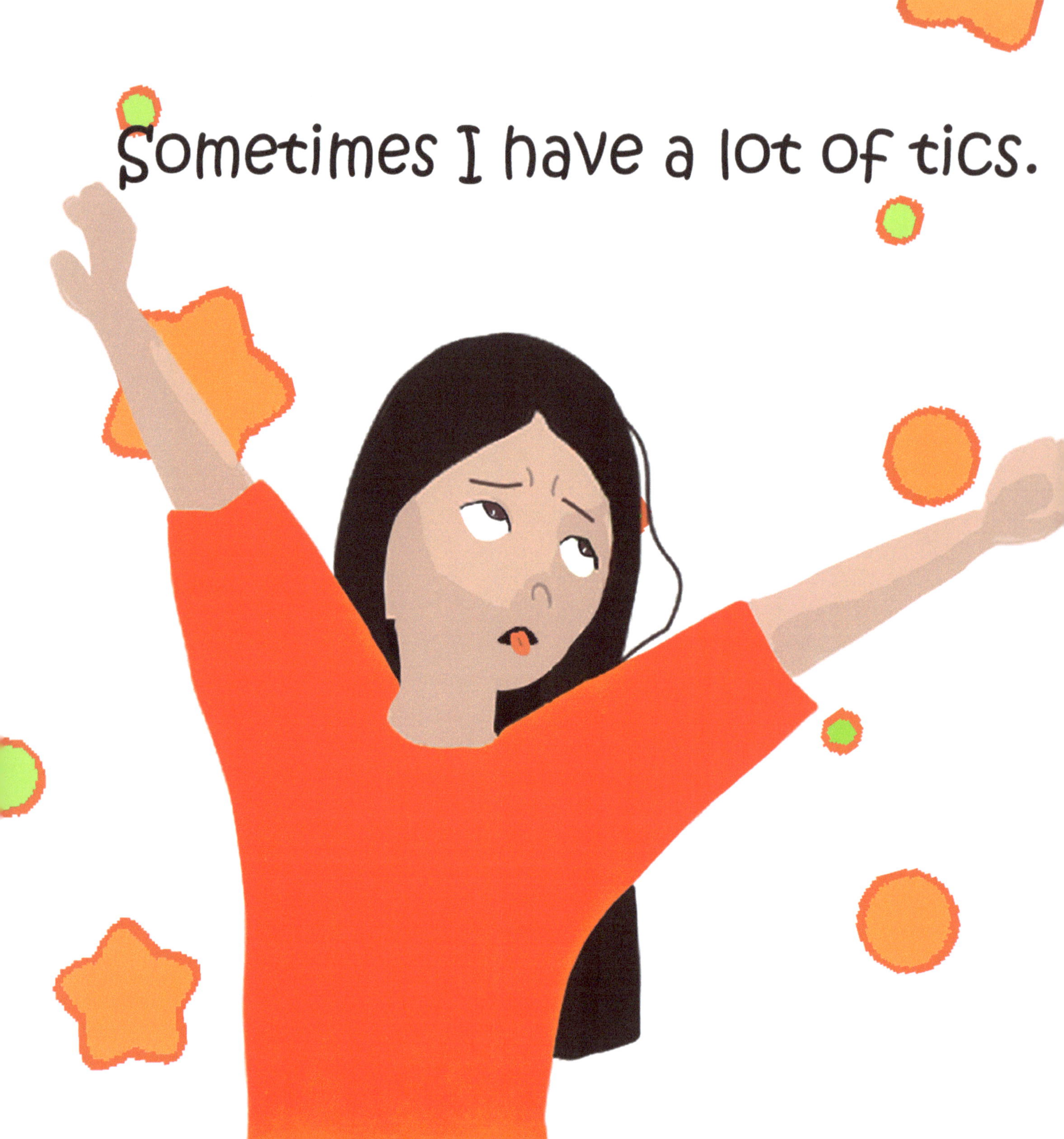

Sometimes I have a lot of tics.

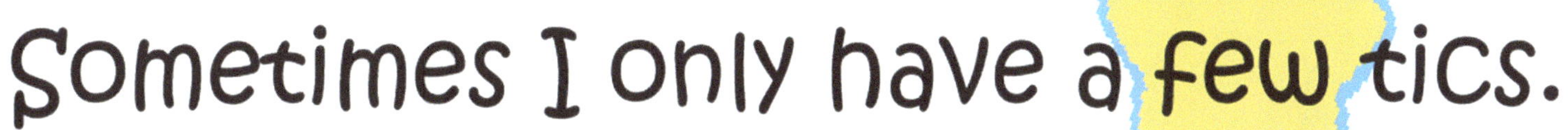
Sometimes I only have a few tics.

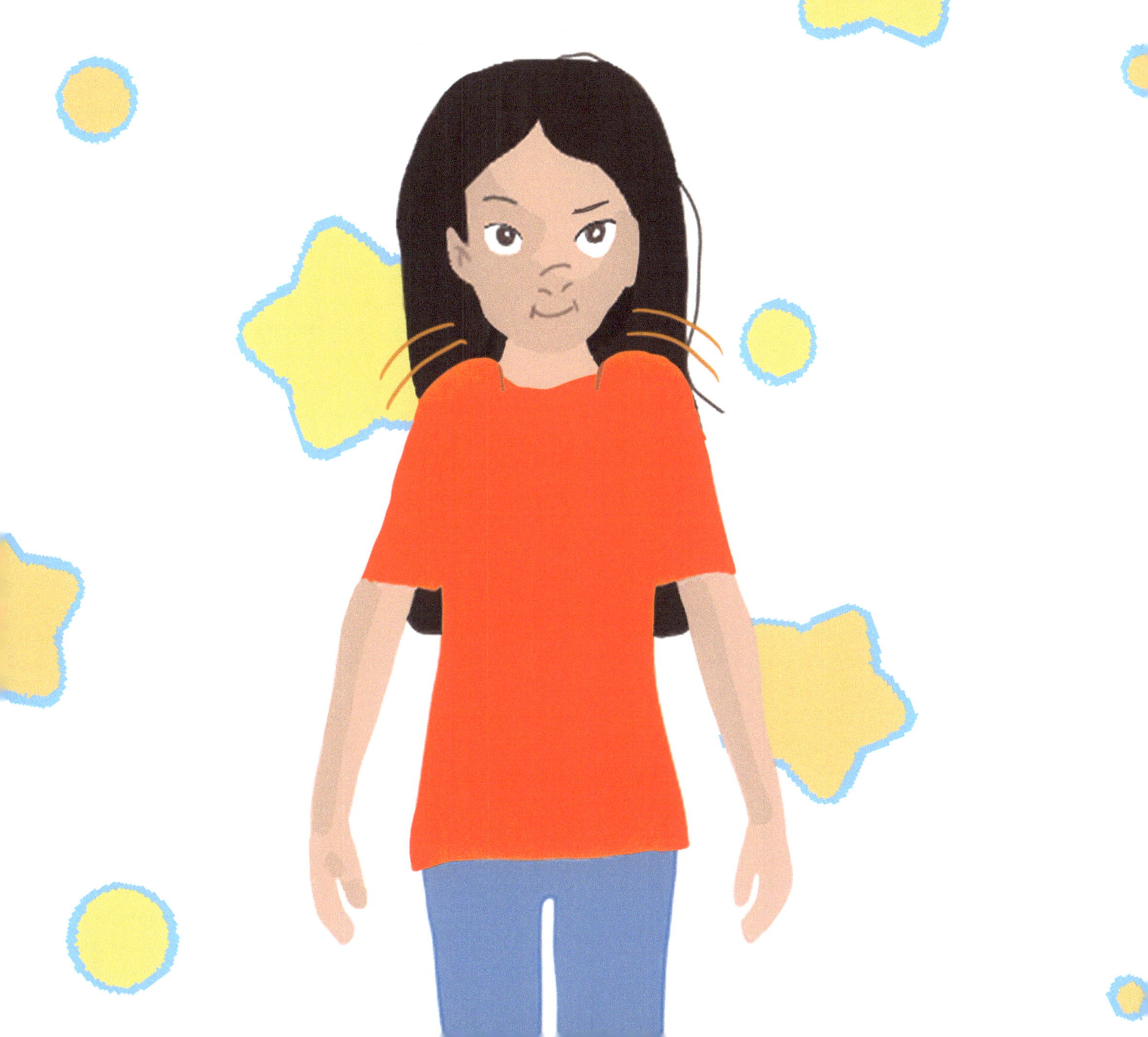

Tics can be bad some days and better on other days. If I'm feeling stressed, anxious or nervous my tics get worse, but if I'm focused on something they calm down some.

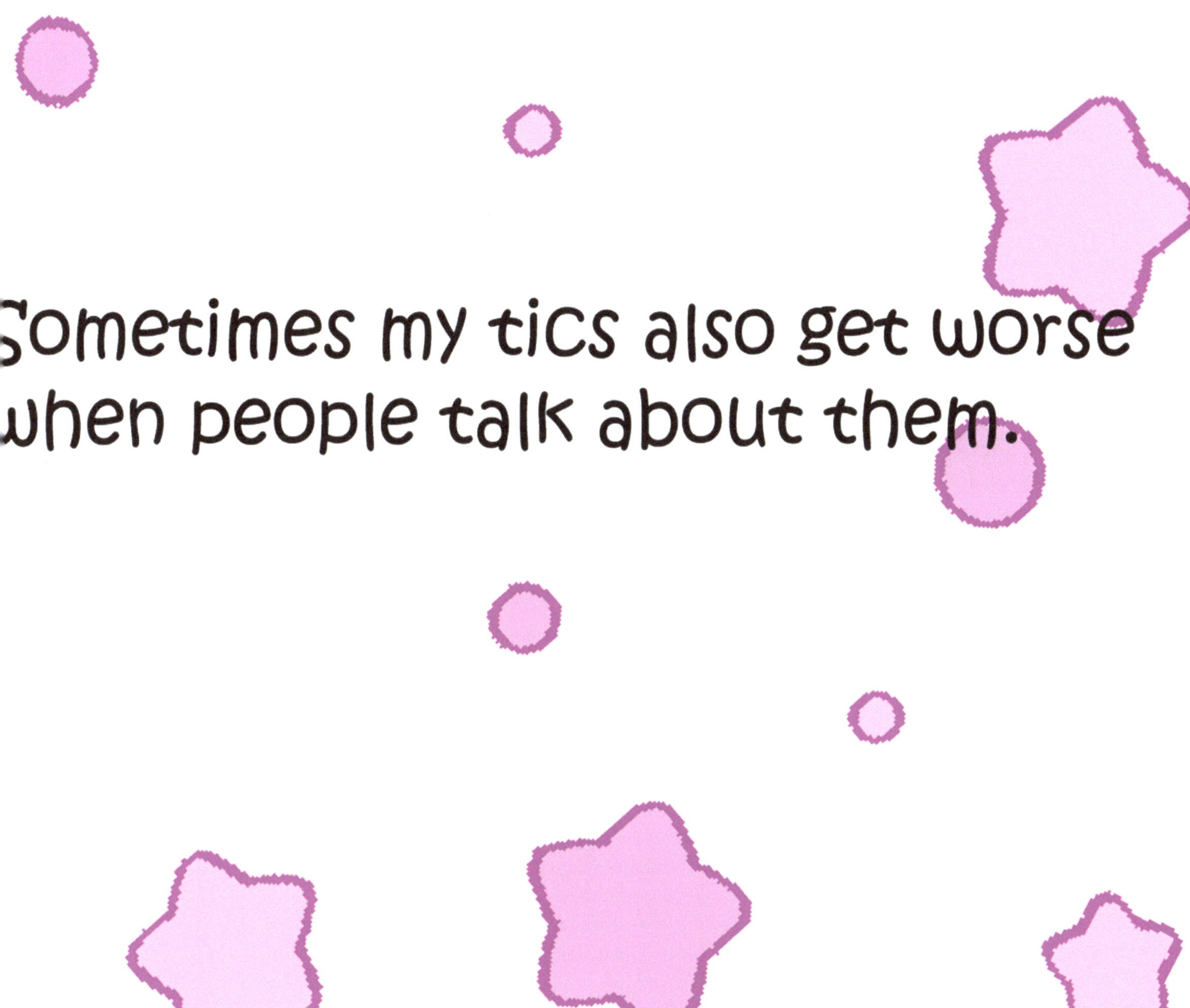

Sometimes my tics also get worse when people talk about them.

When I tic in public sometimes I get weird faces made at me.

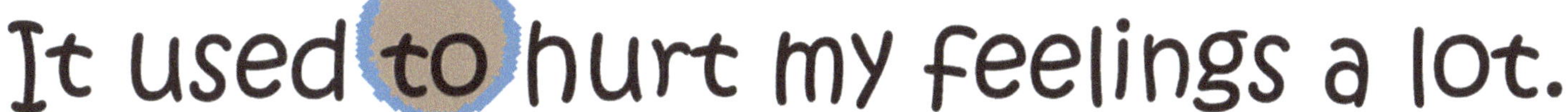

It used to hurt my feelings a lot.

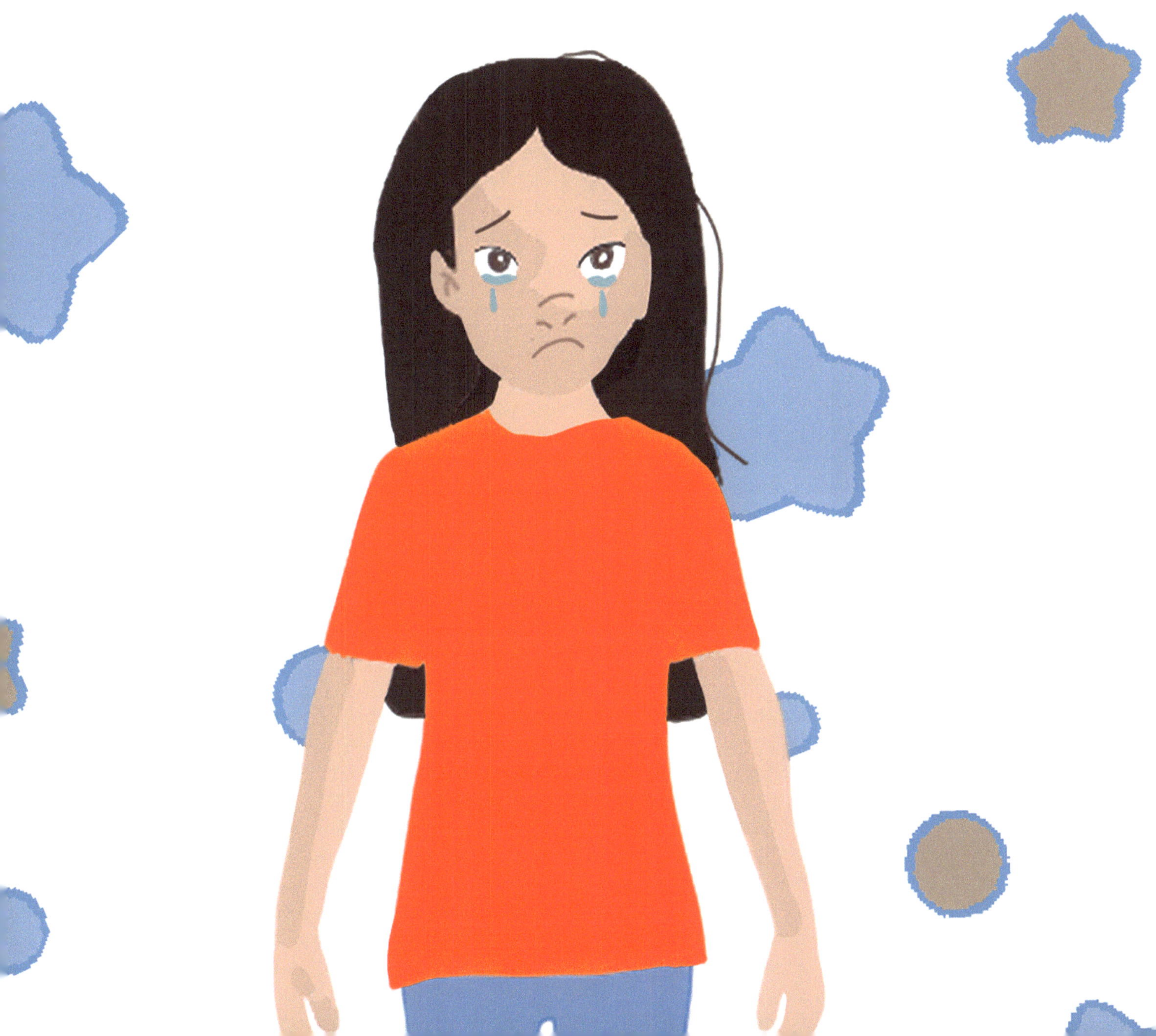

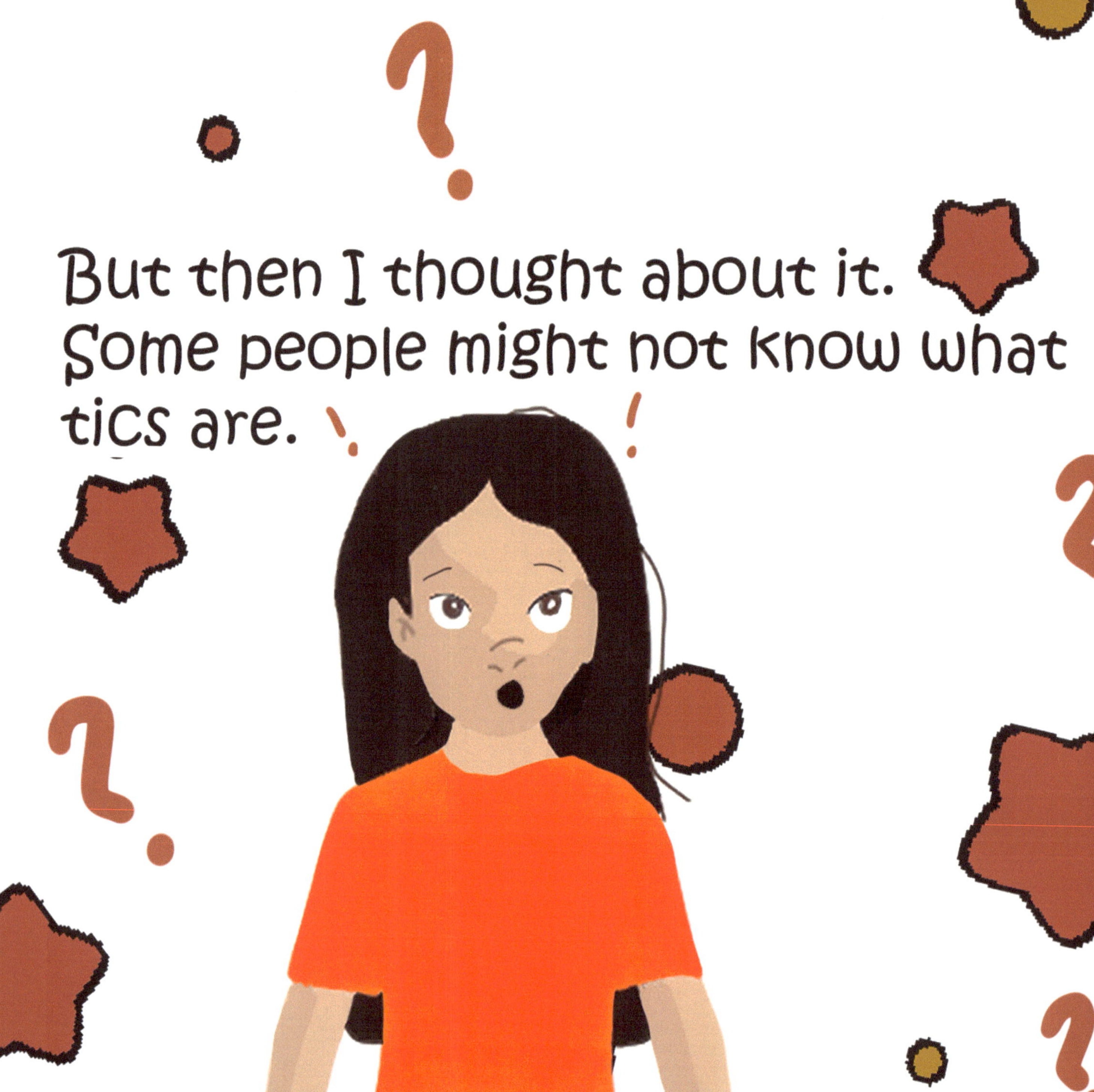

But then I thought about it.
Some people might not know what
tics are.

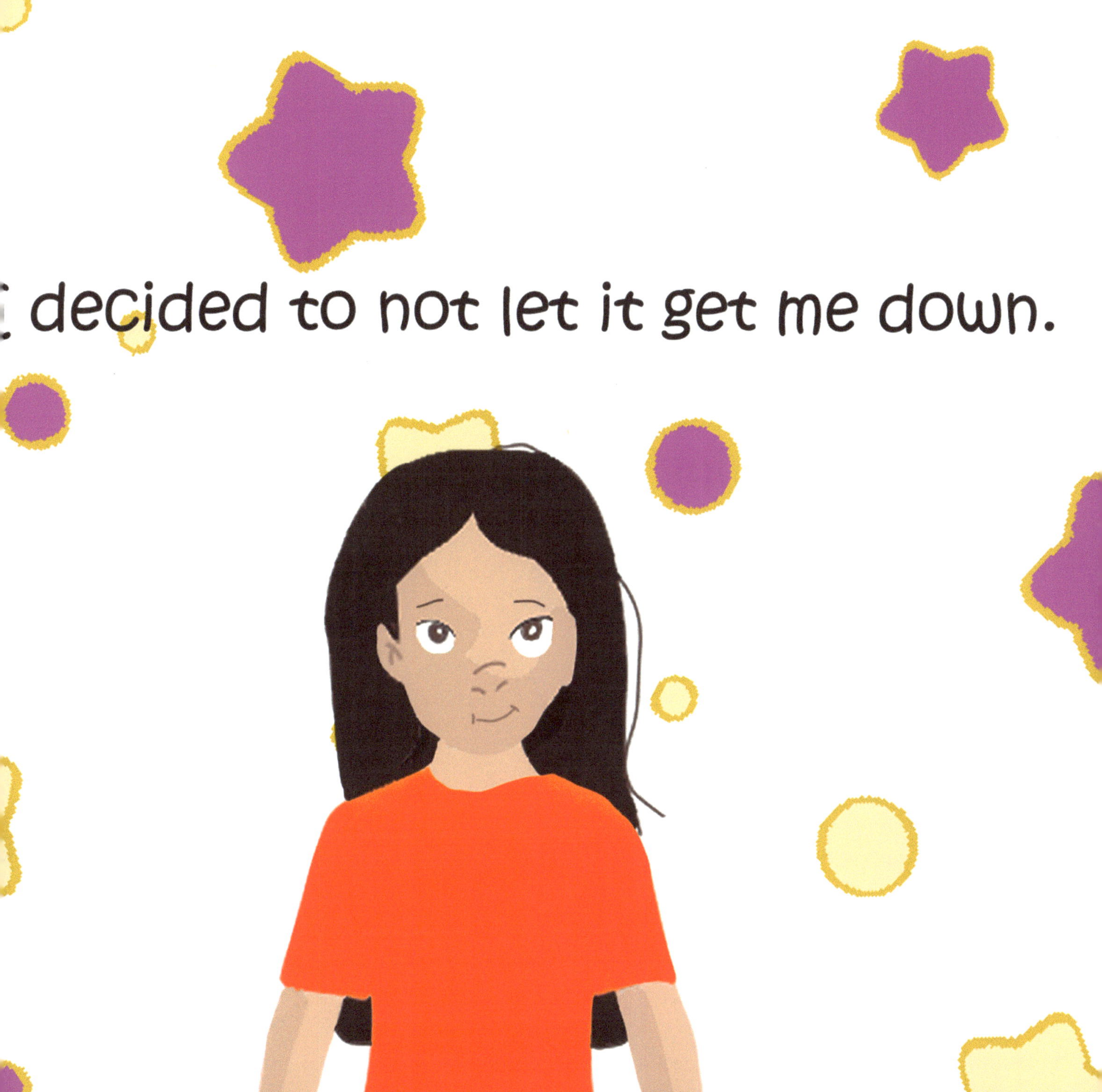

I decided to not let it get me down.

Letting it get me down instead of doing
something to help others understand
about my diagnosis didn't seem like
the right thing to do.

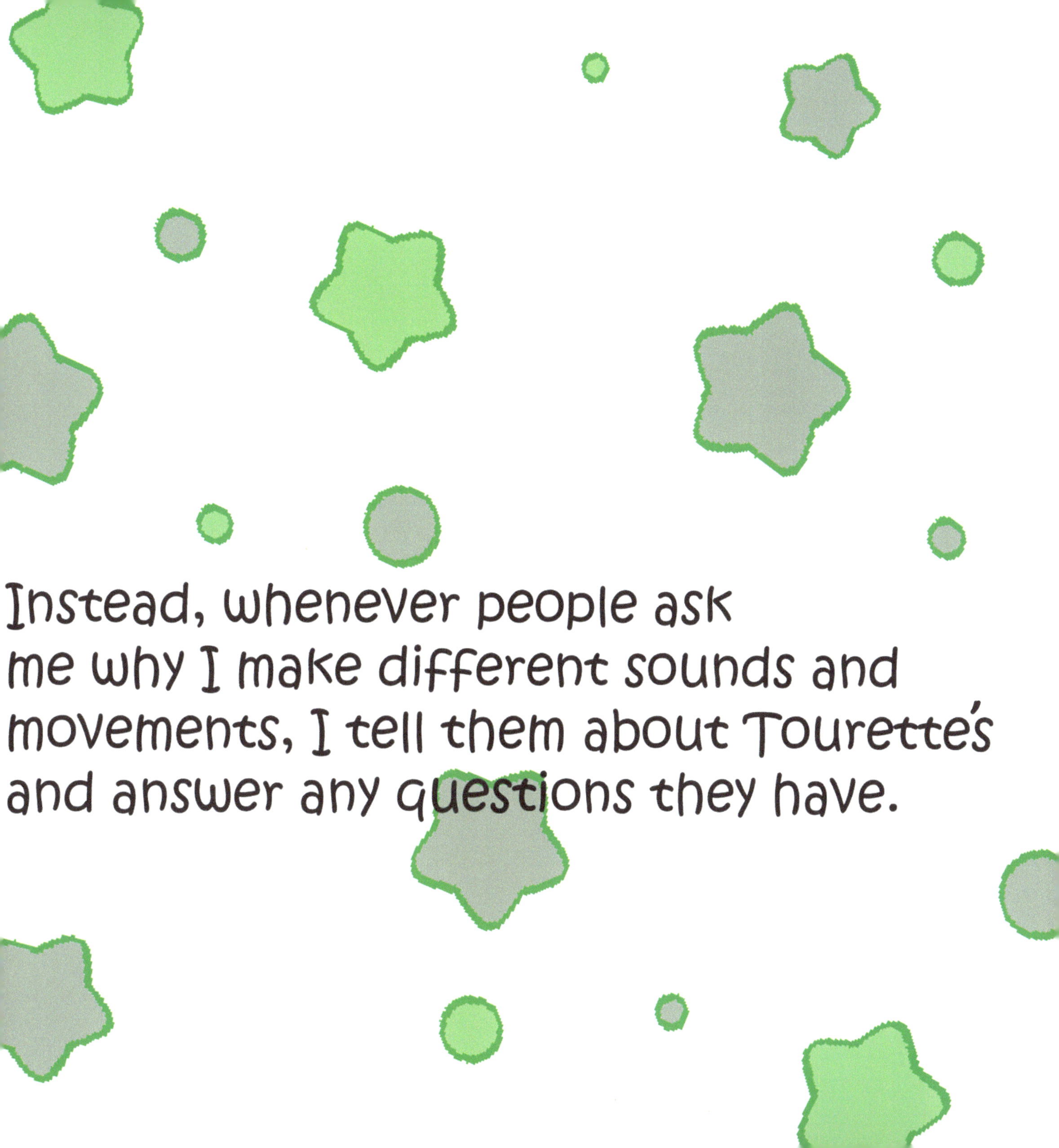
Instead, whenever people ask
me why I make different sounds and
movements, I tell them about Tourette's
and answer any questions they have.

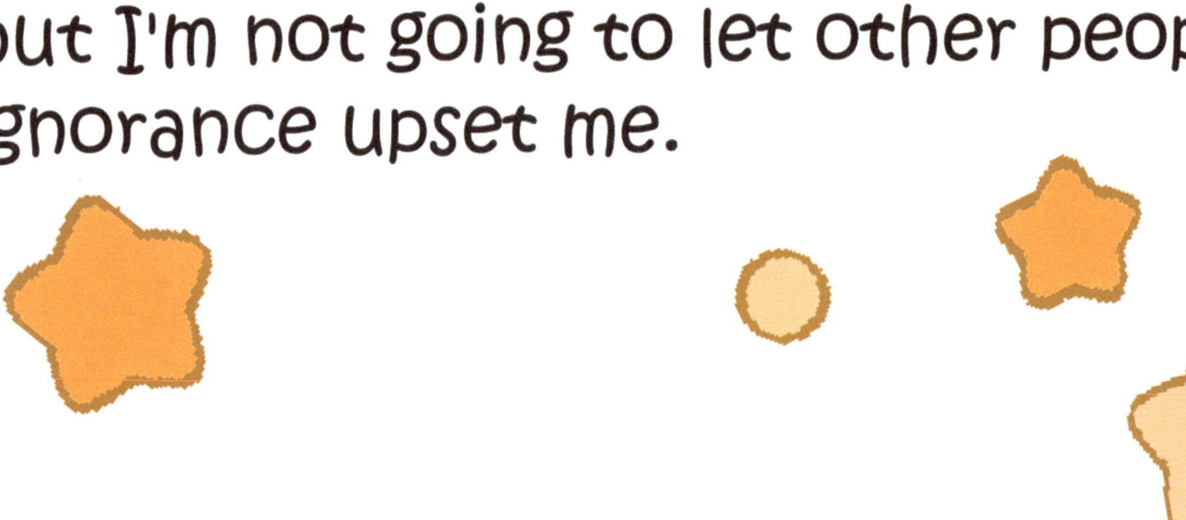

A few times people still didn't understand or would say mean things but I learned to ignore it. It still hurts my feelings sometimes but I'm not going to let other people's ignorance upset me.

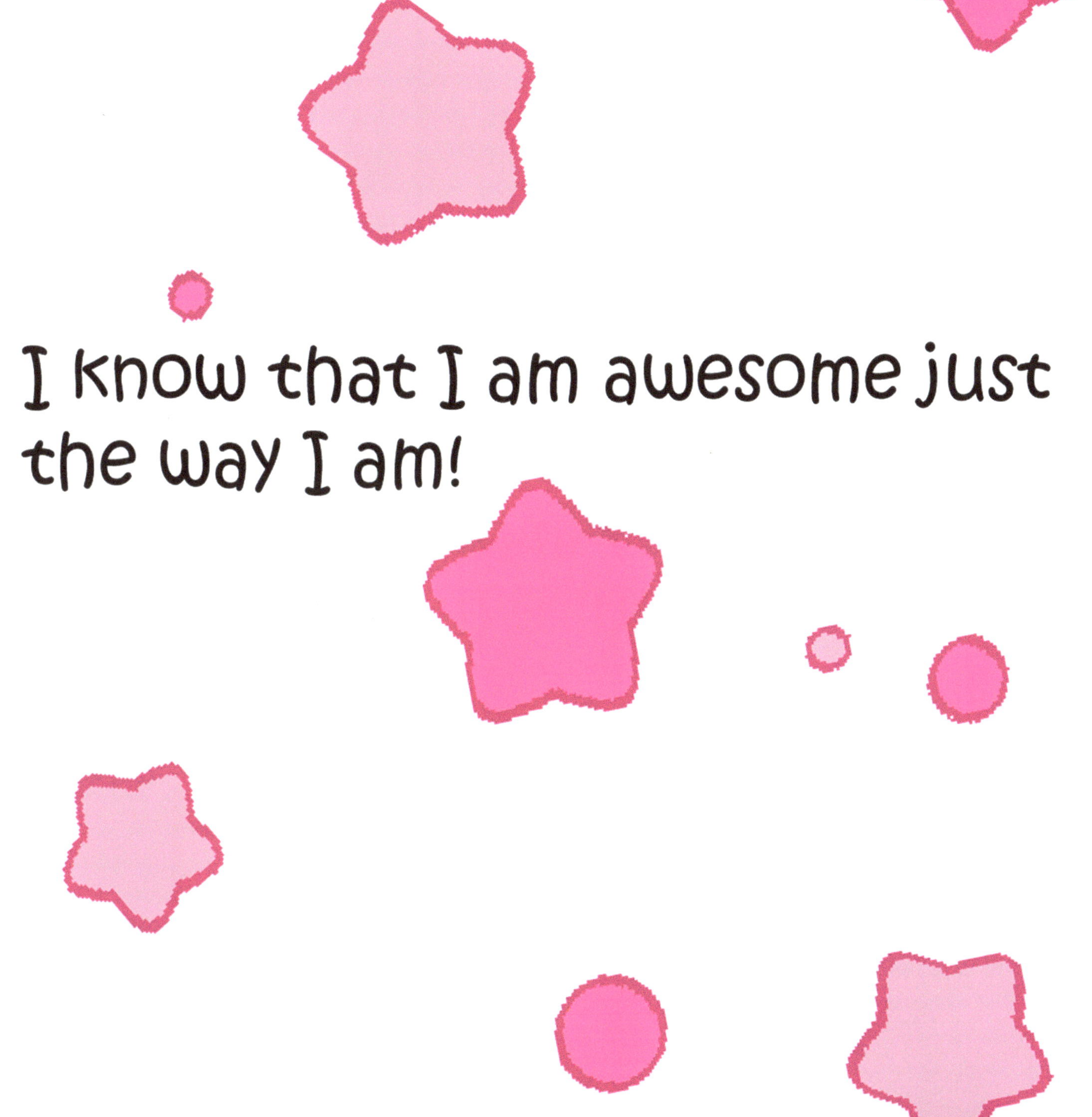
I know that I am awesome just the way I am!

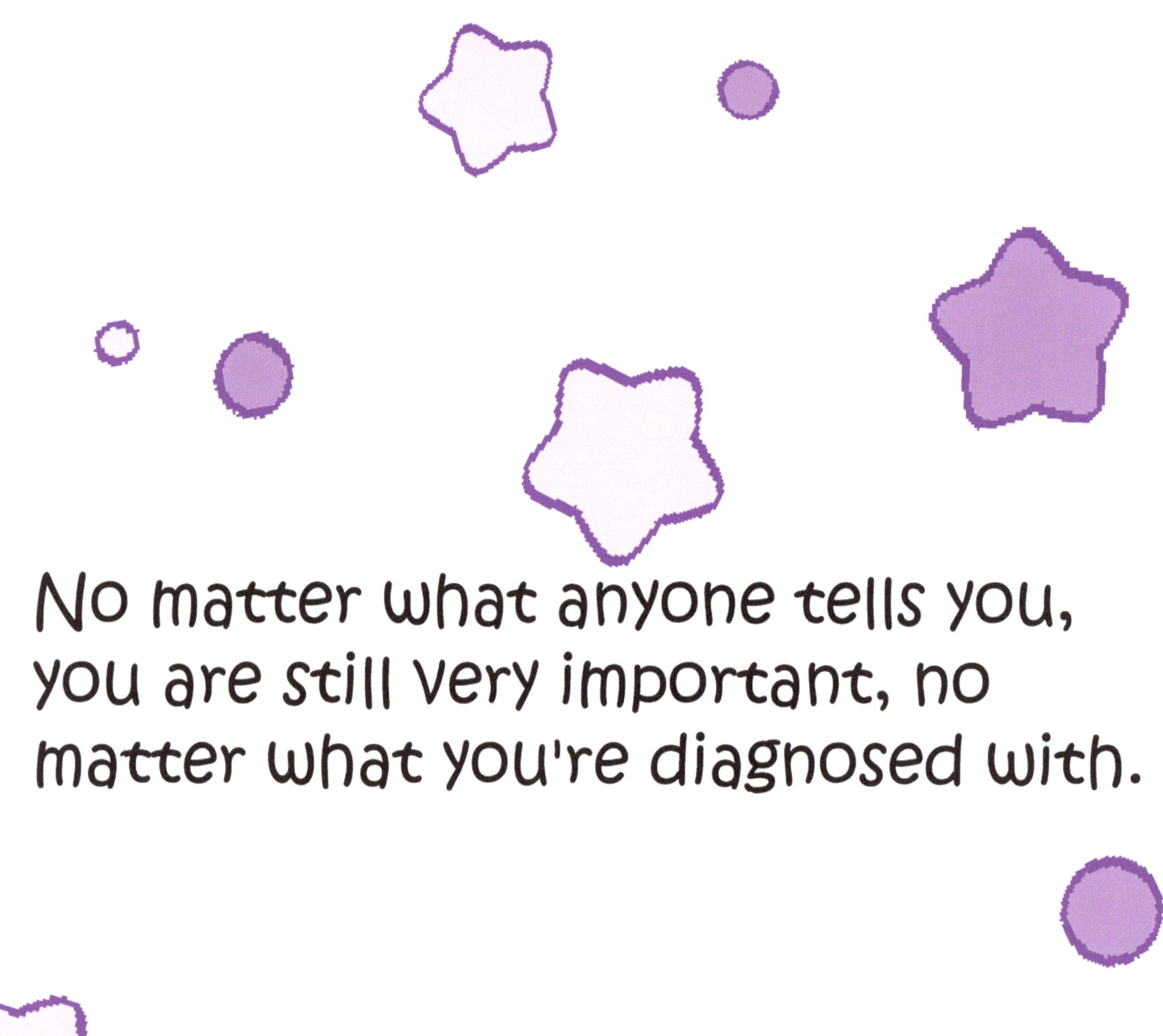

No matter what anyone tells you, you are still very important, no matter what you're diagnosed with.